# FOODS THAT CAN CHANGE ACIDITY LEVEL OF YOUR URINE

## Which Ultimately Affects Your Blood's PH level

JOSEPH THOMPSON

ISBN: 9781728961958
ISBN-13:

# DEDICATION

To My Family Mom, Dad and all my sisters and brothers.

# CONTENTS

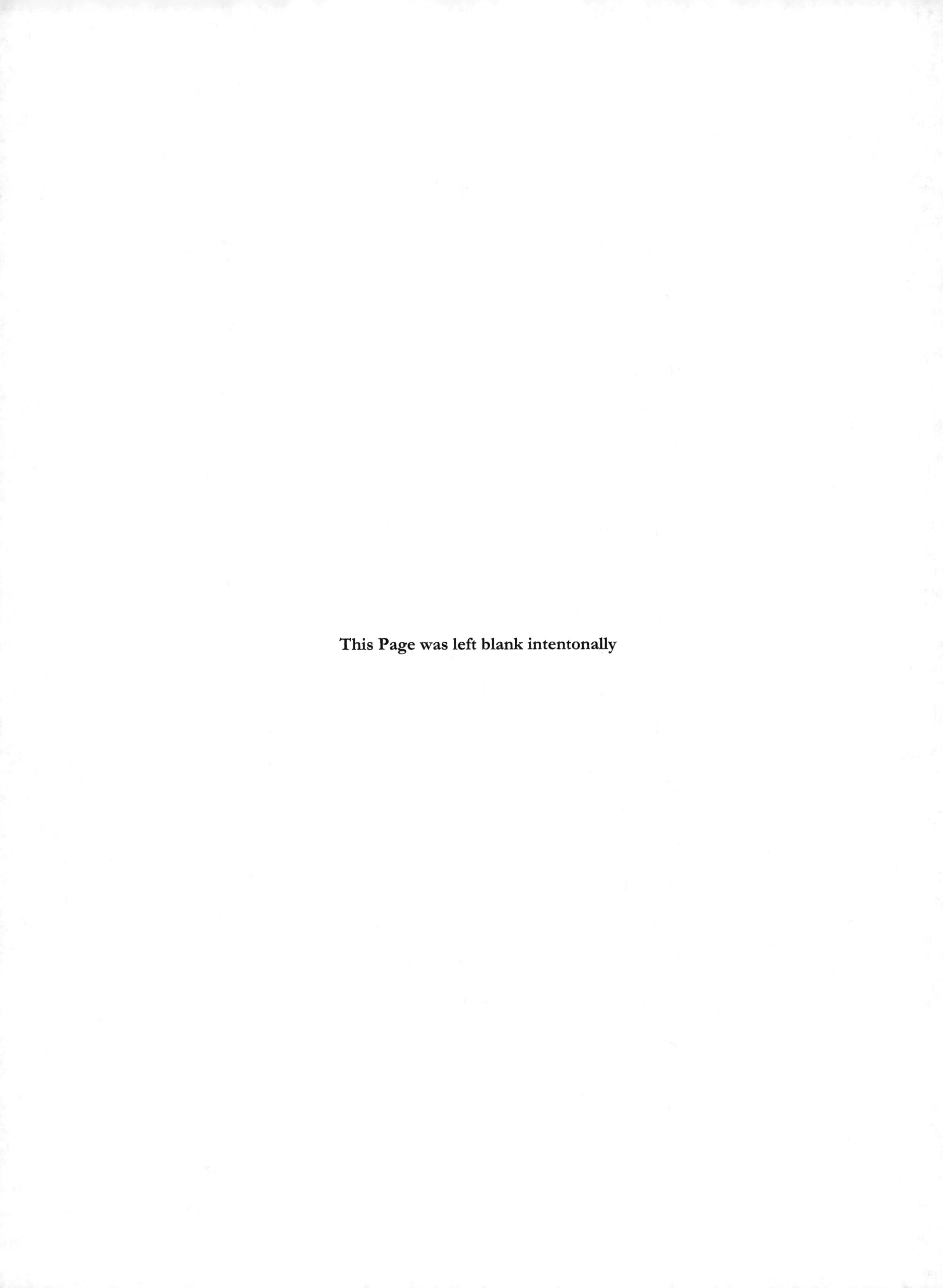

This Page was left blank intentonally

# ACKNOWLEDGMENTS

All New York Public Library for use of computers.

# CHAPTER 1
## ALKALIZING VEGETABLES

Alfalfa

Barley Grass

Beet Greens

Beets

Broccoli

Cabbage

Carrot

Cauliflower

Celery

Chard Greens

Chlorella

Collard Greens

Cucumber

Dandelions

Dulce

Edible Flowers

Eggplant

Fermented Veggies

Garlic

Green Beans

Green Peas

Kale

Kohlrabi

Lettuce

Mushrooms

Mustard Greens

Nightshade Veggies

Onions

Parsnips (high glycemic)

Peas

Peppers

Pumpkin

Radishes

Rutabaga

Sea Veggies

Spinach, green

Spirulina

Sprouts

Sweet Potatoes

Tomatoes

Watercress

Wheat Grass

Wild Greens

# CHAPTER 2
## ALKALIZING ORIENTAL VEGETABLES

Daikon

Dandelion Root

Kombu

Maitake

Nori

Reishi

Shitake

Umeboshi

Wakame

# CHAPTER 3
# ALKALIZING FRUITS

Apple

Apricot

Avocado

Banana (high glycemic)

Berries

Blackberries

Cantaloupe

Cherries, sour

Coconut, fresh

Currants

Dates, dried

Figs, dried

Grapes

Grapefruit

Honeydew Melon

Lemon

Lime

Muskmelons

Nectarine

Orange

Peach

Pear

Pineapple

Raisins

Raspberries

Rhubarb

Strawberries

Tangerine

Tomato

Tropical Fruits

Umeboshi Plums

Watermelon

| ALKALIZING PROTEIN | ALKALIZING SWEETENERS | ALKALIZING SPICES & SEASONINGS |
|---|---|---|
| Almonds | Stevia | Chili Pepper |
| Chestnuts | | Cinnamon |
| Millet | | Curry |
| Tempeh (fermented) | | Ginger |
| Tofu (fermented) | | Herbs (all) |
| Whey Protein Powder | | Miso |
| | | Mustard |
| | | Sea Salt |
| | | Tamari |

# 5 CHAPTER

| ALKALIZING  OTHER | ALKALIZING MINERALS |
| --- | --- |
| Alkaline Antioxidant Water | Calcium: pH 12 |
| Apple Cider Vinegar | Cesium: pH 14 |
| Bee Pollen | Magnesium: pH 9 |
| Fresh Fruit Juice | Potassium: pH 14 |
| Green Juices | Sodium: pH 14 |
| Lecithin Granules | |
| Mineral Water | |
| Molasses, blackstrap | |
| Probiotic Cultures | |
| Soured Dairy Products | |
| Veggie Juices | |

## ACIDIFYING VEGETABLES

Corn

Lentils

Olives

Winter Squash

## ACIDIFYING FRUITS

Blueberries

Canned or Glazed Fruits

Cranberries

Currants

Plums**

Prunes**

## ACIDIFYING GRAINS, GRAIN PRODUCTS

Amaranth

Barley

Bran, oat

Bran, wheat

Bread

Corn

Cornstarch

Crackers, soda

Flour, wheat

Flour, white

Hemp Seed Flour

Kamut, Wheat Germ

Macaroni

Noodles

Oatmeal

Oats (rolled)

Quinoa

Rice (all)

Rice Cakes

Rye

Spaghetti

Spelt

# 7  CHAPTER
## ACIDIC BEANS, LEGUMES DAIRY, NUTS AND OTHER DAIRY

| ACIDIFYING BEANS & LEGUMES | ACIDIFYING DAIRY | ACIDIFYING NUTS & BUTTERS |
|---|---|---|
| Almond Milk | Butter | Cashews |
| Black Beans | Cheese | Legumes |
| Chick Peas | Cheese, Processed | Peanut Butter |
| Green Peas | Ice Cream | Peanuts |
| Kidney Beans | Ice Milk | Pecans |
| Lentils | | Tahini |
| Pinto Beans | | Walnuts |
| Red Beans | | |
| Rice Milk | | |
| Soy Beans | | |
| Soy Milk | | |
| White Beans | | |

# ACIDIFYING ANIMAL PROTEIN

Bacon

Beef

Carp

Clams

Cod

Corned Beef

Fish

Haddock

Lamb

Lobster

Mussels

Organ Meats

Oyster

Pike

Pork

Rabbit

Salmon

Sardines

Sausage

Scallops

Shellfish

Shrimp

Tuna

Turkey

Veal

Venison

# 9 CHAPTER

| ACIDIFYING FATS & OILS | ACIDIFYING SWEETENERS | ACIDIFYING ALCOHOL |
|---|---|---|
| Avocado Oil | Carob | Beer |
| Butter | Corn Syrup | Hard Liquor |
| Canola Oil | Sugar | Spirits |
| Corn Oil | | Wine |
| Flax Oil | | |
| Hemp Seed Oil | | |
| Lard | | |
| Olive Oil | | |
| Safflower Oil | | |
| Sesame Oil | | |
| Sunflower Oil | | |

| ACIDIFYING OTHER FOODS | ACIDIFYING DRUGS & CHEMICALS | ACIDIFYING JUNK FOOD |
| --- | --- | --- |
| Catsup | Aspirin | Beer: pH 2.5 |
| Cocoa | Chemicals | Coca-Cola: pH 2 |
| Coffee | Drugs, Medicinal | Coffee: pH 4 |
| Mustard | Drugs, Psychedelic | |
| Pepper | Herbicides | |
| Soft Drinks | Pesticides | |
| Vinegar | | |

# 11 CHAPTER
# RANKED FOODS: ALKALINE TO ACIDIC

| Extremely Alkaline | Alkaline Forming | Moderately Alkaline |
|---|---|---|
| Lemons, watermelon. | Cantaloupe cayenne celery, dates, figs, kelp, limes, mango, melons, papaya, parsley, seaweeds, seedless grapes (sweet), watercress.<br><br>Asparagus, fruit juices, grapes (sweet), kiwifruit, passionfruit, pears (sweet), pineapple, raisins, umeboshi plums, and vegetable juices. | Apples (sweet), alfalfa sprouts, apricots, avocados, bananas (ripe), currants, dates, figs (fresh), garlic, grapefruit, grapes (less sweet), guavas, herbs (leafy green), lettuce (leafy green), nectarine, peaches (sweet), pears (less sweet), peas (fresh, sweet), pumpkin (sweet), sea salt (vegetable).<br><br>Apples (sour), beans (fresh, green), beets, bell peppers, broccoli, cabbage, carob, cauliflower, ginger (fresh), grapes (sour), lettuce (pale green), oranges, peaches (less sweet), peas (less sweet), potatoes (with skin), pumpkin (less sweet), raspberries, strawberries, squash, sweet Corn (fresh), turnip, vinegar (apple cider). |

## 12 Chapter
## RANKED FOODS: ALKALINE TO ACIDIC

Slightly Alkaline

Almonds, artichokes (Jerusalem), Brussel sprouts, cherries, coconut (fresh), cucumbers, eggplant, honey (raw), leeks, mushrooms, okra, olives (ripe), onions, pickles (homemade), radishes, sea salt, spices, tomatoes (sweet), vinegar (sweet brown rice).

Chestnuts (dry, roasted), egg yolks (soft cooked), essene bread, goat's milk and whey (raw), mayonnaise (homemade), olive oil, sesame seeds (whole), soy beans (dry), soy cheese, soy milk, sprouted grains, tofu, tomatoes (less sweet), and yeast (nutritional flakes).

Neutral

Butter (fresh, unsalted), cream (fresh, raw), cow's milk and whey (raw), margarine, oils (except olive), and yogurt (plain).

Moderately Acidic

Bananas (green), barley (rye), blueberries, bran, butter, cereals (unrefined), cheeses, crackers (unrefined rye, rice and wheat), cranberries, dried beans (mung, adzuki, pinto, kidney, garbanzo), dry coconut, egg whites, eggs whole (cooked hard), fructose, goat's milk (homogenized), honey (pasteurized), ketchup, maple syrup (unprocessed), milk (homogenized).

Molasses (unsulfured and organic), most nuts, mustard, oats (rye, organic), olives (pickled), pasta (whole grain), pastry (whole grain and honey), plums, popcorn (with salt and/or butter), potatoes, prunes, rice (basmati and brown), seeds (pumpkin, sunflower), soy sauce, and wheat bread (sprouted organic).

## 13 CHAPTER
## ALKALINE FORMING FOODS: VEGETABLES

| | |
|---|---|
| Garlic | Mushrooms |
| Asparagus | Mustard Greens |
| Fermented Veggies | Dulce |
| Watercress | Dandelions |
| Beets | Edible Flowers |
| Broccoli | Onions |
| Brussel sprouts | Parsnips (high glycemic) |
| Cabbage | Peas |
| Carrot | Peppers |
| Cauliflower | Pumpkin |
| Celery | Rutabaga |
| Chard | Sea Veggies |
| Chlorella | Spirulina |
| Collard Greens | Sprouts |
| Cucumber | Squashes |
| Eggplant | Alfalfa |
| Kale | Barley Grass |
| Kohlrabi | Wheat Grass |
| Lettuce | |
| Wild Greens | |

# 14 CHAPTER
# ALKALINE FORMING FOODS: FRUITS

Apple

Apricot

Avocado

Banana (high glycemic)

Cantaloupe

Cherries

Currants

Dates & Figs

Grapes

Grapefruit

Lime

Honeydew Melon

Nectarine

Orange

Lemon

Peach

Pear

Pineapple

All Berries

Tangerine

Tomato

Tropical Fruits

Watermelon

# A LIST OF ACID & ALKALINE FORMING FOODS PROTEIN

| | |
|---|---|
| EGGS (POACHED) | FLAX SEEDS |
| WHEY PROTEIN POWDER | PUMPKIN SEEDS |
| COTTAGE CHEESE | TEMPEH (FERMENTED) |
| CHICKEN BREAST | SQUASH SEEDS |
| YOGURT | SUNFLOWER SEEDS |
| ALMONDS | MILLET |
| CHESTNUTS | SPROUTED SEEDS |
| TOFU (FERMENTED) | NUTS |

## OTHER

| | |
|---|---|
| APPLE CIDER VINEGAR | MINERAL WATER |
| BEE POLLEN | ALKALINE ANTIOXIDANT WATER |
| LECITHIN GRANULES | GREEN TEA |
| PROBIOTICS CULTURES | HERBAL TEA |
| GREEN JUICE | DANDELION TEA |
| VEGGIES JUICE | GINSENG TEA |
| FRESH FRUIT JUICE | BANCHI TEA |
| ORGANIC MILK | KOMBUCHA |
| (UNPASTEURIZED) | |

# 16 CHAPTER
# A LIST OF ACID & ALKALINE FORMING SWEETNERS, AND SPICES

| SWEETENERS | SPICES/SEASONINGS | ORIENTAL VEGETABLES |
|---|---|---|
| Stevia | Cinnamon | Maitake |
| Ki Sweet | Curry | Daikon |
|  | Ginger | Dandelion Root |
|  | Mustard | Shitake |
|  | Chili Pepper | Kombu |
|  | Sea Salt | Reishi |
|  | Miso | Nori |
|  | Tamari | Umeboshi |
|  | All Herbs | Wakame |
|  |  | Sea Veggies |

## 17 CHAPTER
## A LIST OF ACID & ALKALINE FORMING FATS, GRAINS AND DIARY

| FATS & OILS | GRAINS | DAIRY |
|---|---|---|
| Avocado Oil | Rice Cakes | Cheese, Cow |
| Canola Oil | Wheat Cakes | Cheese, Goat |
| Corn Oil | Amaranth | Cheese, Processed |
| Hemp Seed Oil | Barley | Cheese, Sheep |
| Flax Oil | Buckwheat | |
| Lard | Corn | |
| Olive Oil | Oats (rolled) | FRUITS |
| Safflower Oil | Quinoa | Cranberries |
| Sesame Oil | Rice (all) | |
| Sunflower Oil | Rye | |
| | Spelt | |
| | Kamut | |
| | Wheat | |
| | Hemp Seed Flour | |

# 18 CHAPTER
# A LIST OF ACID & ALKALINE
# FORMING NUTS, ANIMAL PROTEIN AND PASTA

| NUTS & BUTTERS | ANIMAL PROTEIN | PASTA (WHITE) |
|---|---|---|
| Cashews | Beef | Noodles |
| Brazil Nuts | Carp | Macaroni |
| Peanuts | Clams | Spaghetti |
| Peanut Butter | Fish | |
| Pecans | Lamb | OTHER |
| Tahini | Lobster | Distilled Vinegar |
| Walnuts | Mussels | Wheat Germ |
| Butter | Oyster | Potatoes |
| | Pork | DRUGS & CHEMICALS |
| | Rabbit | Aspartame |
| | Salmon | Chemicals |
| | Shrimp | Drugs, Medicinal |
| | Scallops | Drugs, Psychedelic |
| | Tuna | Pesticides |
| | Turkey | Herbicides |
| | Venison | |

# 19 CHAPTER
## A LIST OF MORE ACID & ALKALINE FORMING FOODS & DRINKS

ALCOHOL

Beer

Spirits

Hard Liquor

Wine

BEANS & LEGUMES

Black Beans

Chick Peas

Green Peas

Kidney Beans

Lentils

Lima Beans

Pinto Beans

Red Beans

Soy Beans

Soy Milk

White Beans

Rice Milk

Almond Milk

## 20 CHAPTER
## LEVELS OF ACID & ALKALINE FORMING FOODS

**Acid Forming Foods**

Vanilla, alcohol, black tea, balsamic vinegar, cow milk, aged cheese, soy cheese, goat milk, game meat, lamb, mutton, boar, elk, shell fish, mollusks, goose, turkey, buckwheat, wheat, spelt, teff, kamut, farina, semolina, white rice, almond oil, sesame oil, safflower oil, tapioca, seitan, tofu, pinto beans, white beans, navy beans, red beans, aduki beans, lima beans, chard, plum, prune and tomatoes.

**Low Acid Forming Foods**

vinegar, cream, butter, goat/sheep cheese, chicken, gelatin, organs, venison, fish, wild duck, triticale, millet, kasha, amaranth, brown rice, pumpkin seed oil, grape seed oil, sunflower oil, pine nuts, canola oil, spinach, fava beans, black-eyed peas, string beans, wax beans, zucchini, chutney, rhubarb, coconut, guava, dry fruit, figs, and dates.

**Moderately Acid Forming Foods**

Nutmeg, coffee, casein, milk protein, cottage cheese, soy milk, pork, veal, bear, mussels, squid, chicken, maize, barley groats, corn, rye, oat bran, pistachio seeds, chestnut oil, lard, pecans, palm kernel oil, green peas, peanuts, snow peas, other legumes, garbanzo beans, cranberry, and pomegranate.

# 21 CHAPTER
## More Ranked Foods: Alkaline (pH) to Acidic (pH)

| Low(pH) | 2 | 3 | 4 | 5 | 6 | 7 | 8 | 9High(pH) |
|---|---|---|---|---|---|---|---|---|
| | | | | | | | | |

**(Ph)5**

5.0  Artificial sweeteners

5.5  Beef, Carbonated soft drinks & fizzy drinks 38, Cigarettes (tailor made), Drugs, Flour (white, wheat) 39, Goat, Lamb, Pastries & cakes from white flour, Pork, Sugar (white) 40

Beer 34, Brown sugar 35, Chicken, Deer, Chocolate, Coffee 36, Custard with white sugar, Jams, Jellies, Liquor 37, Pasta (white), Rabbit, Semolina, Table salt refined and iodized, Tea black, Turkey, Wheat bread, White rice, White vinegar (processed).

**(Ph)6**

6.0  Cigarette tobacco (roll your own), Cream of Wheat (unrefined), Fish, Fruit juices with sugar, Maple syrup (processed), Molasses (sulphured), Pickles (commercial), Breads (refined) of corn, oats, rice & rye, Cereals (refined) eg weetbix, corn flakes, Shellfish, Wheat germ, Whole Wheat foods 32, Wine 33, Yogurt (sweetened)

6.5  Bananas (green), Buckwheat, Cheeses (sharp), Corn & rice breads, Egg whole (cooked hard), Ketchup, Mayonnaise, Oats, Pasta (whole grain), Pastry (wholegrain & honey), Peanuts, Potatoes (with no skins), Popcorn (with salt & butter), Rice (basmati), Rice (brown), Soy sauce (commercial), Tapioca, Wheat bread (sprouted organic)

**(Ph)7**

7.0  Almonds 17, Artichokes (Jerusalem), Barley-Malt (sweetener-Bronner), Brown Rice Syrup, Brussel Sprouts, Cherries, Coconut (fresh), Cucumbers, Egg plant, Honey (raw), Leeks, Miso, Mushrooms, Okra, Olives ripe 18, Onions, Pickles 19, (home made), Radish, Sea salt 20, Spices 21, Taro, Tomatoes (sweet), Vinegar (sweet brown rice), Water Chestnut

Amaranth, Artichoke (globe), Chestnuts (dry roasted), Egg yolks (soft cooked), Essene bread 22, Goat's milk and whey (raw) 23, Horseradish, Mayonnaise (home made), Millet, Olive oil, Quinoa, Rhubarb, Sesame seeds (whole) 24, Soy beans (dry), Soy cheese, Soy milk, Sprouted grains 25, Tempeh, Tofu, Tomatoes (less sweet), Yeast (nutritional flakes)

7.0  Barley malt syrup, Barley, Bran, Cashews, Cereals
(unrefined with honey-fruit-maple syrup), Cornmeal,
Cranberries 30, Fructose, Honey (pasteurized),
Lentils, Macadamias, Maple syrup (unprocessed),
Milk (homogenized) and most processed dairy
products, Molasses (unsulphered organic) 31,
Nutmeg, Mustard, Pistachios, Popcorn & butter
(plain), Rice or wheat crackers (unrefined), Rye
(grain), Rye bread (organic sprouted), Seeds
(pumpkin & sunflower), Walnuts

Blueberries, Brazil nuts, Butter (salted), Cheeses
(mild & crumbly) 28, Crackers (unrefined rye),
Dried beans (mung, adzuki, pinto, kidney,
garbanzo) 29, Dry coconut, Egg whites, Goats
milk (homogenized), Olives (pickled), Pecans,
Plums 30, Prunes 30, Spelt

7.5  Apples (sour), Bamboo shoots, Beans (fresh green),
Beets, Bell Pepper, Broccoli, Cabbage;Cauli, Carob
13, Daikon, Ginger (fresh), Grapes (sour), Kale,
Kohlrabi, Lettuce (pale green), Oranges, Parsnip,
Peaches (less sweet), Peas (less sweet), Potatoes
& skin, Pumpkin (less sweet), Raspberry, Sapote,
Strawberry, Squash 14, Sweet corn (fresh), Tamari
15, Turnip, Vinegar (apple cider) 16

**(Ph)8**

8.0  Apples (sweet), Apricots, Alfalfa sprouts 9,
Arrowroot, Flour 10, Avocados, Bananas (ripe),
Berries, Carrots, Celery, Currants, Dates & figs
(fresh), Garlic 11, Gooseberry, Grapes (less sweet),
Grapefruit, Guavas, Herbs (leafy green), Lettuce
(leafy green), Nectarine, Peaches (sweet), Pears
(less sweet), Peas (fresh sweet), Persimmon,
Pumpkin (sweet), Sea salt (vegetable) 12, Spinach

8.5  Agar Agar 3. Cantaloupe, Cayenne (Capsicum) 4,
Dried dates & figs, Kelp, Karengo, Kudzu root, Limes,
Mango, Melons, Papaya, Parsley 5, Seedless grapes
(sweet), Watercress, Seaweeds
Asparagus 6, Endive, Kiwifruit, Fruit juices 7, Grapes
(sweet), Passion fruit, Pears (sweet), Pineapple,
Raisins, Umeboshi plum, Vegetable juices 8

**(Ph)9**

9.0  Lemons 1, Watermelon 2

www.ingramcontent.com/pod-product-compliance
Lightning Source LLC
Chambersburg PA
CBHW081829250726
48657CB00011B/3531